WHERE WOULD YOU LIKE YOUR NIPPLE?

(Navigating the breast cancer abyss with humor and hope)

By

MACKENZIE CROWNE

Dedication:

For my family and friends, who held my hand, eased my heart, propped me up…and carried my sorry behind when all else failed. You're the best!

Acknowledgements:

Many thanks to talented artist, Lisa Scholder for providing *Open Heart* for the cover image of this work. Lisa has a heart for survivors and is currently body painting breast cancer survivors for a documentation project with "Faces of Courage" providing, at no cost to participants, day outings and overnight camps for women, children and families touched by all cancers and blood disorders. *Open Heart* is part of the "Bodies of Courage" Arts in Medicine Project.

Visit their websites for more information.
LisaScholder.com * Facesofcourage.org * Bodiesofcourage.org

***

Cancer.

Though it's not a four-letter word, it sure conjures up a lot of them. I won't say the first word that popped into my mind, and out of my mouth, when I received the diagnosis of breast cancer — it's a bad word, my mother would be horrified. I *can* tell you it wasn't Whoopee!

Crap. That's like seven letters. My bad.

Many other four-letter words quickly joined that first, shocked sentiment. *Fear, sick, pain, loss, hell, dead...* You get the drift. If you're reading this and have received a similar diagnosis, or know someone who has, I don't want to scare you. You're scared enough already, and have probably experienced many of those words yourself, but, though your fears are justified, I *can* share one four-letter word that trumps all others.

Hope.

Okay, so it took me a little while to get from those nasty words to that one. But I did eventually get there. I'm no longer the same woman I was when I began my journey, and that's not necessarily a bad thing. Sure, I faced some incredibly crappy stuff, but I also learned a lot about myself in the process. Let me tell you, living like you're dying has some unexpected benefits; once you get past the "holy crap" factor.

To do that, I needed to get through the first few weeks. They passed in a haze of doctors' appointments and terror. Shortly after receiving the diagnosis, I met the first of many breast cancer survivors. Suddenly, like pink ribbons during Breast Cancer Awareness Month, survivors were everywhere. They seemed to come out of the woodwork like members of a secret society, calling to me to enter into the fold. But I didn't feel I belonged. I wasn't anything like those women. They danced, victorious, on the other side of an abyss, while I staggered under quiet disbelief.

Their acceptance of such a devastating reality made no sense to me. Here were women who had been where I currently stood, and yet, they seemed so confident and upbeat, almost serene. Honestly, I thought they were nut jobs. I certainly didn't feel like a survivor. I felt like a victim.

A wise person once said, *"Life happens. It's time to pull on your big girl panties and deal with it."*

Big girl panties in place, I took those first, staggering steps toward survival. Somehow, during the last five, life-altering years, I managed to navigate the abyss to join the survivors waiting for me on the other side. The following pages are my personal observations of my odyssey.

I am a survivor. You can be too. Victory is ours.

Chapter One

Find Her An Empty Lap, Fellas!

(Comfort in the midst of chaos)

So, who is Mackenzie? I'm a wife, mother, and grandmother. A daughter, sister, and friend. I'm also a storyteller. I write romance novels—ahem, shameless plug—and until that fateful phone call, I led a charmed life.

Oh, I don't live in a big house or drive the Jaguar XJ I've always lusted after. I've never won the lottery, and the Publisher's Clearing House guy has never shown up at my door with balloons and one of those giant checks. I was never a great beauty, and life with my husband and our two sons more closely resembled one of today's wacky reality shows than yesterday's *Leave It To Beaver*.

Still, I've always considered myself blessed. I have a husband whom I've loved, fought, and laughed with for over a quarter century, and two now-grown sons I genuinely like for the caring men they've become. A beautiful daughter-in-law joined the mix and gave us two spunky grandbabies. Their addition to the family only increased my sense of having it all.

My perception of living a charmed life began in childhood. I'm one of eight kids, and my mom and dad were excellent parents. I woke up every day to the knowledge I was loved.

With so many of us in one household, my parents dealt with just about everything a child could dish out. We saw our share of scrapes and bruises, and the occasional broken bone. We had our disappointments and battled one another occasionally, but none of us ended up in prison for sibling murder.

Remember that scene in *Good Will Hunting* where Will rattles off the names of all his fictitious brothers? I've done that my entire life, but in my case, the names are real. I'm number five in the birth order. My youngest sister, number seven in the count, has a habit of referring to us by birth number. In the interest of privacy in this writing, and because it will give her a laugh, I've done the same.

I have four sisters and three brothers, and can't overstate how much we sincerely like each other—most of the time, anyway.

Growing up, I didn't understand the rarity of my existence. As an adult, I was amazed to discover not all families were like ours. Not everyone grows up with parents who stay together and show their kids how to love and respect one another on a daily basis. We did.

Until recently, the only truly traumatic event in my life was my father's death from leukemia after he'd battled the illness for many years. We still miss him desperately. He was an insurance salesman, and mom was a nurse. We moved several times while I was young, leaving the Midwest for New England. Both my parents came from large families and my childhood was full of love, laughter, and road trips to visit extended family in New York and St. Louis.

My parents genuinely loved people. They collected them like generation X-ers collect electronics. Like happy gypsies, they ran our home with an open door policy. I never knew when I'd walk through the door to find a cousin, a family friend, or a complete stranger—usually a foreign exchange student—ensconced in my bedroom.

Raised as we were instilled a certain amount of confidence in my sibs and me, along with an ability to adjust to new situations. It was a surprise to no one that we all scattered across the country when it came time to raise our own families. Somehow, those of us who married managed to choose spouses that fit into the family like siblings; we like them as friends and love them as family. Despite the miles separating us, we're all still close and get together as often as possible.

I met my husband at eighteen. We married five years later and had our first son several years after that. A weeklong trip to Arizona, where my husband grew up, was all it took to seal my fate. One look out the window of the plane as we landed in Phoenix and I knew I was home.

It took some time to work out the logistics, but we eventually made the move to the southwest, where our second son was born. Though exciting, those first years in Phoenix weren't easy. New in town, and home with a four year-old and a newborn, I'd left behind my career, my family, and a large group of friends.

With so many siblings, you learn early on to be assertive or be trampled under the crush of personalities. Consequently, like my parents, I could speak to anyone and I, too, became a collector of people. But suddenly, for the first time in my life, I found it difficult to cultivate new friendships.

I felt as if I were stuck inside a weird, invisible bubble of isolation. The experience left me more than a little frustrated. Though raised in a Christian home, I'd never really given the whole 'God' thing a lot of thought. Stranded inside the bubble, that changed. Years later, I realized being separated from my family and friends left a void. God was more than happy to fill the hole.

I'm happy to report my friendless state was short-lived. I met some incredible women during those early years in Phoenix, who remain close friends to this day. To my joy, I also discovered a loving Father who knew my wants and needs and was there, just there, whenever life turned messy.

Now, don't get nervous. My purpose for writing about my experience isn't to proselytize. That's not my job. My purpose is to share how I went from victim to survivor, and my faith played a key role in my journey.

The word "God" has many connotations for people. My perception of God is that of ultimate parent, a benevolent father. As a parent myself, I want only the best for my children. I do whatever is humanly possible to help them succeed. When the situation arises where nothing I can do will help, I'm simply there for them, giving them the confidence and the comfort of my love.

For me, God is like that, only on steroids. He's so much better at parenting than I will ever be. Over the past five years, I've scrambled into His lap countless times, spiritually speaking of course, and was comforted, confident in His love.

I consider my faith a huge advantage in my breast cancer battle. I can't imagine facing mastectomies, reconstruction, chemotherapy, and radiation with only myself and the medical profession to look to for confidence of a complete recovery.

It's not my intention to belittle the many doctors, nurses, and other health care professionals I've become acquainted with along the way. I've met some extremely talented, very dedicated people. But even as well trained as they all are, what they do is not an exact science. They couldn't give me assurances. The best they could do was increase the odds of my survival. I needed assurances.

I found them in my faith.

The battle against breast cancer is debilitating and draining. Where will *you* find the confidence to forge ahead? Where will you find comfort?

Chapter Two

Infiltrating Lobular Carcinoma

(Now, there's a mouthful)

The tarnishing of my charmed life began with a phone call. Oh, not that one from my doctor. Did I mention I am not the only member of the family who has battled this senseless disease? No? Well, apparently there are spots of breast cancer algae in the old gene pool. One moment, life was bustling along the way it was supposed to, and the next, one of my sisters, number six in the count, was diagnosed with breast cancer.

That call shook my family's world.

If you haven't discovered it already, you'll learn there are many reactions to the word cancer. My family's reactions to Six's news ran the gamut from fear to hope.

My take on her diagnosis was colored by my memories of a close friend's breast cancer experience seven years earlier. I'd supported my friend by supplying meals when needed and transportation for a follow up appointment or two, but I hadn't been there to witness the day-to-day trials of her treatment.

I'd avoided the experience, the same way I'd avoided the day-to-day details of Dad's illness and treatment. To my shame, I found the process too painful to watch, so I looked away as much as possible, grateful others in my group of friends were comfortable enough to be there in her darkest hours, as my family had been in Dad's.

Consequently, the memories from my friend's bout with breast cancer were intense, but limited. I remembered only that she had faced her diagnosis and treatment with grace and strength, and though she was very sick for a long while, she's been cancer free for years and is healthy and happy.

So, while my heart broke for Six, I didn't immediately panic. In hindsight, I should have been peeing my pants at what she was facing, and as I was soon to discover, what I would face.

When someone is going through an illness, any illness, those around them tend to be more conscious of the indicators and preventive measures. Suddenly, the many women in my family were doing self-exams. Can you imagine my shock when I discovered a lump? A large lump?

I was due for a mammogram at the time. I'd been having them regularly for years, but I no longer did self-exams as a rule. Remember that game you played as a child, where you threw a beanbag across a distance to drop through a hole in a section of wood? My breasts had the consistency of one of those beanbags. I'd found a number of questionable lumps over the years, all of which had proven to be simple cystic clusters. Having had enough of the pattern of panic and relief, I quit doing the self-exams and relied completely on annual mammograms. As it turned out, that was *not* one of my finer decisions.

When the phone call came from Six, I hadn't yet made my yearly appointment, so I can't say for sure if I would have had a mammogram any time soon. Someone or something would have eventually reminded me it was time to see the doc, but knowing me, it might have been months later. I can't say for certain my sister's diagnosis saved my life, but considering I now had a lump over three centimeters in size that hadn't been there the year before, it's plausible.

So, thanks, Six. This makes up for all those times you raided my closet and jewelry box when we were teenagers.

While I waited to learn if I was dealing with cancer or just another cluster in my beanbag-breasts, Six already had no doubt. Infiltrating Lobular Carcinoma. That's what the doctors called it. A month later, I read the same words on *my* pathology report.

Growing up in a family of eight kids with a fifteen-year age span, we were categorized into three different age groups; the older kids, myself and Six, and the younger ones. Because Six is only two years younger than me, we spent a lot of time together in the same environment. We slept in the same bed as little girls and the same room for most of our teenage years. We attended school together and enjoyed many of the same extra-curricular activities.

When you and a sibling are diagnosed with the same cancer within a month of each other, you start wondering if environment might be the cause. Was there lead in the paint of the hallway dormer where our bed was located when we were little, or toxic chemicals in the water of that swimming pool where we camped when we were in our teens? Personally, I think there was something in the soap we used to scrub the kitchen floor every Saturday morning when Six and I were assigned that unfair chore.

I'm telling you, Six, we should have protested harder over that injustice.

While I am an artsy, big picture kind of girl, Six has always been detail oriented. When Dad got sick and was going through treatment, Six researched each new phase while I accepted Dad's calm explanations of his diagnosis and treatment plans and didn't dig any deeper for details. "Ignorance is bliss" was my motto.

Six and I followed that same pattern when we were diagnosed. Having no interest in gaining a medical degree on a supersonic schedule, I was content to take the facts given me by the docs. In contrast, Six researched like a maniac. I decided I liked my style a whole lot better, when her discoveries scared the crap out of both of us.

Sharing my feelings and concerns with a sister I love was a tremendous comfort, but despite that silver lining, I sincerely hope your sisters are healthy and you never experience what we did. There are many women out there battling this disease at any given time. I suggest you find one or more of them to speak to. Your doctor or the staff at the hospital can hook you up with a support group. In fact, they'll probably suggest it first.

Six's choice of surgery was a bilateral mastectomy with immediate reconstruction. Her results came back with the best possible outcome under the circumstances; stage one breast cancer with no spreading to the lymph nodes. Hell, yeah! Go, Six! No chemotherapy or radiation necessary. Long-term hormone therapy was prescribed.

She came through the surgery like a champ and began the process of healing. An infection after surgery slowed down the process a bit, but through it all, her faith remained steady. She was an inspiration to me as I marched through the process of finding and talking to the doctors who would perform my bilateral mastectomy and treatments.

I've never been one of those people who could quote a specific scripture that would bring peace for a specific problem. I'm still not. My brain just isn't wired that way—I have a hard enough time remembering my cell phone number. But in that amazing way God works, both Six and I discovered we had each been directed to the same scripture.

Psalm 91.

In its' entirety, the scripture speaks of doing battle and coming out victorious while under the cover of His protection. For me it was all about Psalm 91:4.

He will cover you with His feathers, and under His wings, you will find refuge.

God has given me many feathers in the form of my family and friends. They were there to cover me while I walked this walk. My hope is that you find the same healing refuge throughout your battle.

Chapter Three

I'm On Cancer Vacation.

(Fiddle-dee-dee)

I began a journal in those first days after diagnosis. As a writer, I suppose that was a natural thing for me to do, but I'd never kept one before. The benefits of the exercise surprised me. Like an intense therapy for my psyche, I found the daily focus helped me deal with the wild swing of emotions I experienced.

The practice came about completely by accident. The day after the biopsy, my husband and I went to Rocky Point, Mexico with several friends. I love the beach, so a lawn chair in the sand was the perfect place to wait for the results. One afternoon, everyone else took a ride to town and I found myself alone, sitting in my chair under the canopy we had erected and gazing out at the Gulf of Mexico.

Normally I would have my laptop with me in such a situation, but I was currently battling a nasty case of writer's block, a circumstance I'd been suffering since my dad decided he'd battled leukemia long enough, and went on to a better place.

But, that's another story. Where was I? Oh, yes…

I'd been too stunned to cry up to that point, but I missed Dad so much at that moment, the dam cracked. Before I knew it, I was weeping. I felt like an idiot, and figured I'd better do something before the locals had me locked up as a crazy person.

I mean, really! Who weeps on a gorgeous beach?

I found an old notebook in our RV, turned to a blank page, and began to write. My format? A letter to Dad. An hour later, I had written four pages. It was the beginning of my journal and I continued the format throughout treatment.

Each day, several times a day, I would sit down and write to Dad. Talking to him about my fears and concerns was a tremendously calming exercise. As a newly diagnosed breast cancer patient, I felt healthy. Yet the doctors had scheduled one test after another. The MRI, the MUGA, the PET, the EKG. No wonder my emotions were all over the place.

Keeping a journal also had an unexpected benefit. Reading back over my entries one day in those early weeks, I noticed my nearly complete absorption in my diagnosis. It was as if my real life had all but disappeared. In its place was an unacceptable existence. My words documented the thoughts and fears of a victim, a woman with a dark present and bleak future. Externally, I waged battle; choosing the most aggressive of treatments while internally, I seemed to be embracing defeat.

In contrast, the few positive exceptions interspersed throughout the dark entries in my journal shone like bright beacons of light. I was drawn to those exceptions. They were glimpses into the soul of the woman I used to be, before the diagnosis paralyzed me. Disgusted with myself, I made an effort to find more of those moments; like my wonder at the rainbow off my back patio one morning, or the hummingbird that visited the feeder several times a day, or my laughter at some silly comment my granddaughter made.

It was a turning point for me. Focusing on the little blips of joy life delivered, I began to claw my way back from the dark.

I know what you're thinking. Really, Mac? You're telling me to look for rainbows, hummingbirds, and silly comments from a toddler? I'm facing having a chunk of my breast removed, or the whole of it, and having toxic chemicals shot through my veins until I'm so ill I can hardly stand.

Yes, you are, and I'm the first to agree, that sucks. But if you're going to beat breast cancer, treatment is an inescapable fact. There's no getting around it, and no matter what protocol is prescribed, it won't be pleasant. The next year at least will be jammed full of cancer related appointments, constantly reminding you of your diagnosis. That's reality and most of it will be out of your control.

The cancer battle can easily become a vortex, sucking you in until nothing else exists. It's debilitating and demoralizing, and human nature being what it is, it's very easy to let your diagnosis define you. But by definition, this is a battle. I didn't want to be defined by 'my' cancer. I wanted to defeat it. I wanted the cancer gone.

It may seem insignificant to focus on the flight of a hummingbird in the midst of mastectomies and toxic treatments, but amazingly, doing so proved to be my first tentative foray toward the other side of the abyss, toward victory. Focusing on the world outside the vortex reminded me there was a whole existence out there that had nothing to do with cancer. Actively grasping at those little blips of joy during the worst hours of my experience, allowed me to take the first steps toward rejoining the world of the living.

Though that process sounds simple, it wasn't easy. I'd recognized my slide into the vortex and was determined not to return there. The trouble was I still had to deal with the day-to-day challenges of cancer. In an effort to keep myself sane, I mentally set aside those challenges as often as possible. I think of the practice as slipping into Scarlett O'Hara mode.

"I can't think about that right now," Scarlett said. "If I do, I'll go crazy. I'll think about that tomorrow."

Oh yeah, Scarlett, I know the feeling. I was Scarlett so often in the weeks leading up to surgery I may as well have been wearing a dress made of drapes. I think I even started to speak with a southern accent.

On those days my calendar didn't include any cancer related appointments, I handed future stresses off to God, and considered myself on cancer vacation.

Thank you, God. And thank you, Scarlett. You rock!

Chapter Four

I Promise, I'm Not Going To Die.

(Keeping the channels of communication open)

The phone rang on the afternoon I returned home from my escape to the beach and I read the name of my gynecologist's office on the caller ID. I'd been waiting for days for the results of the biopsy, but suddenly I developed a raging case of phone fear. That moment was one of those times in life when you want to know and don't want to know at the same. Taking a deep breath, I answered the call.

I guess it takes a while for something that huge to sink in because I felt calm when I set the phone down.

"Was that them?" my husband asked.

"Yes."

"And?"

"It's cancer."

I don't recall his reaction. My body and mind seemed to have switched to automatic. I'd been in the process of heading out to our RV to return some bedding that had been removed to wash when the phone rang. Without another word, I went out to the RV and made up the bed.

The next few days are a blur. The only thing I remember with clarity is making the call to my sisters several hours later. Our family is big on conference calls, but this was one I wasn't all that interested in joining. Two, Six, and Seven all sat silently while I informed them of the results. Six immediately began asking technical questions I couldn't answer, while Seven cried, and Two tried to calm us all down.

Honestly, once I knew the diagnosis, I wasn't all that scared. I'd watched my friend battle her way back and I'd do the same. I was more disappointed than anything and although I knew it was a ridiculous thing to be feeling, I hated having to admit I was sick. I cringed at the way people looked at me when I shared the diagnosis with them. I could see that flash of panic in my friends' eyes before they sucked it up and asked what they could do to help.

Once I'd been diagnosed, there were a million details and decisions to be worked out, and I fell into a pattern that kept me somewhat grounded. My calendar was my focus for those next few weeks. I took everything step-by-step, doctor's appointment by doctor's appointment.

The day I met with the surgeon to decide what course to take, my sister-in-law, Eight's wife, we'll call her Eight-A, came with me. My nerves jangled as we sat in the waiting room. With Six's research in mind, as well as information from several of my nurse friends, I had a general idea of what I would probably decide, but seeing the surgeon suddenly made it all real.

Just before my name was called, I happened to look down at the small table beside me. There, sitting all by itself, instead of the usual magazines you'd expect to find in a doctor's waiting room, was a bible. One of the prayers my sisters and I had been praying was that God would lead me to the right hands to perform the surgeries that were surely ahead of me, and to the right minds for any treatment that followed. I walked back to the examination room with a lighter heart.

The surgeon was an older man, possibly late sixties and soft-spoken. He sat down and picked up my chart. Eight-A waited with pen and paper in hand to take notes.

"So, the results were negative," he said evenly, "though the lump will still need to be removed."

For a stunned moment I just sat there, thinking it had all been a horrible mistake. My heart began pounding in my chest. The astonished hope in Eight-A's eyes suggested she was thinking the same thing. Now, details are not my strong suit, and medical terms never will be, but out of my mouth came the diagnosis I'd been given without even having to think of the unfamiliar terms.

"They told me it was an Infiltrating Lobular Carcinoma," I said slowly.

The surgeon's gray brows jumped together in confusion and he began flipping through the pages in my chart. When he got to the third page and I saw the comprehension on his face, I knew all bets were off. The top two pages were the diagnosis for the second and third lumps they had looked at—bean bags remember?—neither of which were cancerous. The third page held the damning diagnosis.

When he looked at me again, I wanted to lie back on the examination table and cry.

I didn't.

I felt strangely detached as he took me through the surgical options and the possible treatments I would need afterwards. He explained that with Infiltrating Lobular Carcinoma, the possibility of developing cancer in the unaffected breast sometime in the future was high. Although he insisted the choice was up to me, he seemed to be leading me toward removing both breasts in a bilateral mastectomy. Eight-A thought so too. Since that was the course of action I was leaning toward to begin with, it wasn't much of a shock. I had no interest in going through this again. I wanted the cancer gone. I felt as if a foreign enemy had invaded my body and if I was going to war, I wanted to go in with my biggest guns blazing. Nothing less than a complete rout would do in my mind.

I left his office with a tentative surgery date set for two weeks out and a referral for a plastic surgeon to perform the reconstruction I would begin immediately.

I bawled like a baby when I got home.

As a parent, thoughts of your children are heavy on your mind when you receive a diagnosis such as this. You think to yourself, if the worst happens, what will become of my kids? How will my death affect their lives? How will they cope? It ticked me off that I even asked those questions, if only in my own mind, but I'm human. No matter how positive a person you are, or how much faith you have, the doubts sneak in occasionally like a thief in the night. I'm so thankful I had God's lap in those moments.

Like everyone else, both of my boys handled the news differently. Our oldest son hasn't lived with us for years, but is close by. His wife is very close to me and wanted to know everything, as soon as I received new information. More often than not, she'd be waiting at my house when I'd return from seeing yet another doctor, to discuss and support the myriad of decisions I needed to make. She was a great sounding board and kept my son apprised of each step as it came.

Our second son was in his senior year of high school at the time and busy with the theater productions he was involved in. He's something of a ham, a comedian, and a joy to have around. Living in our home, he heard a lot of what was being discussed, but never asked any questions. I was caught up in my own issues and didn't think to sit him down and reassure him.

The first inkling that I may need to do that came with the phone bill for October. Six-hundred dollars for text messages in the month following my diagnosis was a fairly strong indicator he needed to talk to someone. I did just that—after I'd paid the bill. From that point on, I followed Dad's example from his leukemia battle and gave them all updates on what procedures were planned and why. I thought that was enough.

I'd never missed any of the productions at the high school when our son was performing. It's a hoot to see your kid up there on stage, even when he's playing the evil dentist from *Little Shop of Horrors*. Unfortunately, the production of *The Princess Bride* was scheduled to open the day of my surgery. My son arranged for me to be there for the dress rehearsal the night before. I sat in the audience with the adult volunteers and got to see my baby as another villain in his role as Prince Humperdink.

The experience was very special to me, and quite poignant, especially when the theater director opened the show, explaining that one of his seniors wanted to say a few words before they got started. Breathing became difficult with my heart lodged in my throat as my son stepped to center stage. My six-foot-four baby stood there in the spotlight and announced that the night's performance was dedicated to his mom, who was having surgery the next day.

Then he started to cry.

God, I can't tell you what that did to me. I rose to my feet as he stepped off the stage to pull me into his strong, young arms. We stood there together, rocking back and forth, my frightened baby and me.

"I'm scared, Mom," he whispered.

"Don't be," I whispered back. "I'm not going to die. I promise. It's going to be okay."

Despite the tears we shared that evening, that moment with my son is one of those blips of joy I think are so important. I don't tell my family and friends I love them often enough. I told my son that night, and it was sweet!

From then on, I tried to keep the channels of communication open, which wasn't easy. Quite often, I was having a hard enough time dealing with the next step myself, without having to put it into words for my loved ones. I learned however, that those around me were struggling with what and how much to ask. They didn't want to make things harder for me by asking a lot of questions, but they were dealing with their own fears and needed to know what was happening.

Ask your loved ones how much they want to know and then tell them. You'll save them from fear of the unknown and yourself from feeling guilty that they are more scared than they need to be.

If you ask my sons, they'll tell you I've gone from keeping the details to myself, to sharing too many of them. It's amazing how quickly a mother uttering the word *nipple* will send grown men running from the room.

The memory of that day still makes me laugh.

Chapter Five

We Can't All Be Princesses.

(Someone has to clap as I go by)

I have a group of girlfriends. I say that and know you're thinking, *Oh, Mac has some friends*. Wrong. When I say I have a group of girlfriends, what I mean is, I spend as much of my free time as possible with a group of incredible women who are as close to me as my sisters. Think best friend times ten. We've known each other since our kids were little, sharing juice and cookies at long ago playgroups.

Once a month we get together to play bunko, a horrible little game of dice. I hate the game personally, but the exceptional company keeps me going back. We also spend time together on the beach in Mexico, or at the sand dunes in California, or in front of a fire pit on a cool winter evening. Our gatherings are typical, with our husbands or significant others in one clump, making manly noises, and we girls in another, sipping wine and solving the world's problems.

One of the girls has a cabin on the Mogollon Rim northeast of Phoenix. A couple of times every summer, my girlfriends and I head up the hill for a weekend full of fresh air, food and fun. Those weekends are the ultimate in girlfriend therapy.

I love our time at the cabin. We sit on the deck, talking and laughing with the wind through the trees as background music. I even have my own comfy chair. My girlfriends tease me about never leaving the deck, but they do it just to razz me. I may be the princess they call me, but I've been known to chop a piece of wood or gather twigs for the fire pit on occasion. No one would call me a nature girl, but over the years, I've gotten much more comfortable hanging out in the middle of the woods—where bears live! I've yet to see one, but if I ever do, I can guarantee you, I won't be leaving the deck again.

We'd been to the cabin several times that summer and fall, including once shortly after I'd discovered the lump. Scheduled to see my gynecologist the following Monday morning, I was playing things pretty close to the vest. I'd decided not to scare the girls until I knew something concrete. Years ago, our friend who'd battled breast cancer made a comment none of us have ever forgotten.

"One in ten women will be diagnosed with breast cancer," she said shortly after beginning treatment. "I've taken it for the group. The rest of you are in the clear."

In the years following, those odds have increased to one in eight, and at the time, I was afraid I was going to be the one to fulfill the new numbers. By the time we returned to the cabin the last time that fall, my fear had become fact.

The weekend prior to my scheduled surgery, we packed enough food for an army and enough liquor to open our own bar, and headed up the hill. We spent three days huddled by a constant fire, alternating between tears and laughter. More often than not, we experienced both at the same time.

I posted several entries to my journal that weekend:

11/12/07...10am
Hey Dad,
Still here at the cabin with the girls. It's been good in so many ways. Being with them is always a blessing. Despite being a maniac myself these days, I can see their concern and their sense of helplessness, and I'm humbled they've put their own lives on hold for a few days to hold my hand. It dawned on me this morning that this weekend isn't just another trip to the cabin; it is an organized effort on their part to keep my mind occupied while I tick off the moments to Thursday. It never even crossed my mind that I would need that, but it crossed theirs, and like the pushy broads they are, they did something about it.

Do they know how much that means to me? I hope so, because I could never find the words to express my gratitude, even if I wasn't aware of the fact that with this group of incredible women, no thanks are necessary.

Don't tell anyone, but I'm not feeling as brave as I thought I was. Now that surgery is imminent, I just don't want to do it. I know I don't have a choice; not a real one anyway. I could simply say, I'm not doing that, but since I literally can't live with the consequences of that choice, it's not an option.

So, I need to find peace with what's coming. I wish I could go to sleep today and wake up next week. Since that's not an option either, I will continue to ask God to bring me to a place of ease before Thursday morning. Do you think you could do a little whispering in the right ear up there and help me out with that? Love you ... Miss you.

That weekend with my girlfriends will forever be one of the most bittersweet memories I have of them. Although I was too caught up in my own fears and emotions at the time, I now realize it couldn't have been a comfortable time for any of them. They didn't have to invest themselves so completely in getting me through those last fear filled days. The time would have passed without their having to lift a finger. They could have stayed home and avoided the emotional wrenching the weekend ultimately delivered. But because of who they are and because we are a unit, they stood elbow to elbow to form a solid wall of support. Their gentle hands were there to keep me from sliding into a pit of despair.

And their support didn't end with that weekend. My friends helped me in so many ways over the course of treatment, from holding my husband's hand during surgery, to shaving my head when I began to lose my hair during chemo. They fed my family when I was too sick to think of food, and sat in for me to cheer on my son in his starring role in the high school's production of Grease.

I did, however, put my foot down when my girlfriends offered to come clean my house. The mushrooms growing in my toilets were mine, after all, and I didn't want anyone else harvesting them.

I know how lucky I am to have so many incredible women in my life, but every once in a while it's good to be reminded. My girlfriends may tease me occasionally, asking where I've left my tiara, but they are the real royal ones.

My heroines in heels.

Throughout my battle, the people I love had to stand by helplessly while I went through surgery and treatment, and all the nasty things that came along with them. I had to force myself to let my friends help and felt embarrassed each time they did. But it didn't take me long to learn that assisting where they could not only benefited me, it allowed my loved ones to feel they were doing something, anything, to get us through the worst of the process.

This diagnosis will test not only you, but your family and friends as well. Keep that in mind when those around you don't know what to say or do. Like you, they're doing the best they can.

Chapter Six

Honey, Can You Help Me With The Drainage Tubes?

(Waking up cancer free and flat-chested)

Surgery day dawned as one of those perfect mornings in Phoenix. Fall is my favorite time of the year in the southwest. The weather is perfect, but don't tell anyone. There are too many people living here already.

I remember feeling amazingly calm the night before. In Scarlett mode, I didn't dwell on what would happen in the morning. I had just one bad moment when my husband and I climbed into bed that night and he turned to me. I realized this was the last time I would be making love with my husband as a woman with natural breasts. It's impossible to know what having reconstructed breasts will be like, before you have them, but I knew my body would never be the same.

My husband has had to deal with his own emotions throughout my illness and yet, like the strong man he is, he's never wavered. He had to have been frightened as well that night, but when I explained the reason for my dismay, he held me and told me everything would be okay.

"Whatever you look like when all is said and done," he said, "You'll still be the woman I love."

I'm blessed, I tell you.

My brother-in-law took the day off to wait with my husband, and my survivor friend planned to be there as well. By the time I emerged from surgery, so many of my friends and family had converged on the hospital, the staff had to move them to a larger waiting room. The recovery room nurse grinned, informing me that I had my own personal cheering squad crowding the halls. From what they tell me, I missed a good time.

I hate when that happens.

With breast cancer, a concern is that the cancer will spread to the lymph nodes. Several hours before surgery, my surgeon ordered a Lymphoscintigraphy test. As it was explained to me, a radioactive dye would be injected in through my nipple and over the course of several hours, the dye would follow the trail of cancerous cells and indicate any infected nodes.

All I can say about that test is...hmm. Actually, I can't say what I'd like to about that test—Mom would wash my mouth out with soap. I can only wonder if any men have ever had this test done, because if they had, you can bet your ass someone would have found a way to make it less painful.

Beyond the pain was anger. I'd nursed my babies with those breasts and shared the pleasure of my female body with the man I love. It ticked me off that the last sensation I would feel in my nipple was pain, instead of pleasure.

Once that lovely test was done, I had several hours to wait while the dye did its work. I used the time to write in my journal. I won't share the private thoughts I put into words for the ones I love. They are personal and belong to others, but it helped to know that if the unthinkable happened, and I had some freak reaction to the heavy anesthesia I was facing, my friends and family would know my last thoughts were of them.

Ick. That sounds so morbid, doesn't it? Hey, I was under sedation. That's my story and I'm sticking to it.

The morning seemed interminable, but eventually I was wheeled into surgery. The next thing I knew, I awoke to an iron band of fire wrapped around my chest. I had the impression of moving and opened my eyes to see the lights of a hospital hallway whizzing by. My husband was there, holding my hand and walking along side me.

Once settled in a private room, the face of one of my girlfriends suddenly appeared in my field of vision.

"How are you feeling?" she asked.

"I feel like I have a flaming elephant on my chest," I answered. At least I think that was my answer. If it wasn't, it should have been.

It's good to have nurses as friends when you're having major surgery. Like a five foot-two nurse-general, my friend marched from the room and saw to it I received something for the pain immediately. I learned several things in the next few hours, the least of which was that a morphine drip makes me deathly ill. Ugh, vomitorium! Let me tell you, throwing up is massively freaky when you've just had most of your chest surgically removed. I also learned that hospital staff don't comply with the natural tendencies of the greater population when it comes to nocturnal habits. By the time the sun came up, I was convinced a memo had been sent out, requiring every nurse in the facility visit my room.

Other than being poked, prodded, and asked how I was feeling, I don't remember much of my twelve-hour hospital stay following my surgery—Don't *even* get me started on the concept of drive-thru mastectomies. The next cognizant memory I have is of coming home and settling on the couch.

The next few days are a blur of discomfort, but before long, I was beginning to feel a bit more like myself—minus boobs. Don't get me wrong, a bilateral mastectomy is no fun, but within a week, I was feeling pretty good, considering.

I woke from surgery wearing what I came to call my Scuba Steve vest. Bright blue and made of a thick, slightly stretchy material, that ugly vest kept the bandages where they belonged and supported the drainage tubes dangling from my chest like gaudy, yard sale earrings. I have to tell you, those drainage tubes were sick. Thankfully, my husband isn't squeamish because I could hardly stand to look at them. Having tubes hanging from your chest, that need draining every couple of hours is just wrong. My husband never complained once, however. He simply helped me clean them out and zipped me back into my Scuba Steve gear.

I'd say those drainage tubes qualified as one of those 'worse' moments in the 'For Better or Worse' vow.

Usually, my family and I spend Thanksgiving week camping and riding the dunes in California. Since that was out of the question, my husband and I accepted an invitation to join my nurse-general friend and her family in San Diego. "You can recover just as easily in our suite," she insisted. I felt like I was on a 'make a wish' trip when we checked into the Four Seasons.

I wandered all over San Diego in my Scuba Steve vest, sore but happy to have the cancer gone from me. When I'd found the lump, I was a healthy, forty-seven year-old woman who just happened to have breast cancer. A week after surgery, I felt like a healthy forty-seven year-old woman who just happened to have had her breasts removed.

I'd come through the surgery well, but the cancer had spread to four lymph nodes. Though I felt healthy, we knew surgery alone wouldn't be all the treatment I'd need if I was going to beat cancer. I had a week and a half before I had to face what awaited me, so—can you say Scarlett? I went on cancer vacation and had a ball in San Diego.

Chapter Seven

I'm Here For Chemo.

(But, not by choice)

With the results back from surgery, I was given the diagnosis of stage three-breast cancer. According to my surgeon, chemotherapy and radiation were the most likely treatments I would face. The exact protocol would come from the oncologist. It was time to find one.

Having friends in the medical industry helps when you're looking for a doctor. Within days, I had two names with appointments scheduled for consultation. Both were women and their offices were near my home. I saw the most sought after of the two first. Thinking I was prepared, that I had already heard the worst when given the diagnosis, I asked my younger son to drive me to the first consultation, and then had him wait in the lobby.

A tiny, pixie-like woman with a commander-in-chief attitude entered the examination room. Looking around the empty cubicle, she commented that I hadn't brought anyone with me. That should have warned me of what was to come, but of course, it didn't. I explained that my son was in the waiting room, but I didn't want him coming in. In retrospect, I should have used one of my lifelines and called a friend. The next thirty minutes were the most emotionally excruciating of my life.

I didn't cry when she laid out the numbers, though I wanted to. Actually, I wanted to curl up in a ball on the floor, stick my fingers in my ears and chant, la la la, I can't hear you! But I'm a grown woman. That would have been bad form.

A twenty-four percent chance of survival was the first number she gave me and to tell the truth, nothing much registered after that. Immediate chemo, followed by radiation, and then hormone therapy was her prescription. With that plan of action, she gave me a final number. A fifty-six percent chance of survival sounded better than twenty-four to my numbed brain, but it was still a crappy number. I walked out of her office, collected my son, and went home. I was on the phone with Two before the front door slammed shut.

Okay, so those numbers were nasty, but those were just the medical profession's numbers. I am a child of the Great Healer. He has His own plan and His own set of numbers for me, and after a few minutes of conversation to calm me down, I relaxed in that knowledge.

I saw the second oncologist the next day. I brought along a friend as I should have the day before, and heard pretty much the same thing, but I had already heard the worst and I'd already made my decision. The first doc had an aggressive, no-nonsense philosophy. I saw her as a tiny, special ops commando for my own personal war. I'd found my cancer doc.

12/3/07...9:30am
Hi, Dad. Today was a red-letter day for my personal record book. I've just been asked the most ridiculous question of my life. When would I like to start chemo? Hello! Never! But it looks like the thirteenth is the day, as long as all the other tests and the port are done by then. I'm finding some moments in life are a real bitch.

The next few days were so busy I barely had time to be scared, and I was still at the scared stage. Dad had been through chemo, as had my friend, so I knew it was going to be awful. It's an odd thing, to say okay to something you know is going to be so debilitating. It kept crossing my mind that I was an adult, I could just say no. No one could *make* me do this thing. But there was never any question that I would go through with it. With the decision made, I cut my hair short in preparation of losing it, and checked into the hospital to have a port catheter inserted into my chest, where it remained for the four months of chemotherapy treatment.

Several days later, Eight-A showed up unexpectedly at about ten in the morning. I was in my kitchen. She called out to me, saying she had something she needed to drop off. I looked in the living room to find Two standing at my front door. Being so far away from your sisters when you are as close as we are is always difficult, but having them so far away when I needed them most was a hardship, for them as well as me. It makes me tear up now to think of it. I was so glad to see her.

I'd mentioned to one of my girlfriends that instead of wearing a wig or scarves once I lost my hair, I planned to buy a few hats. Two had flown in from Dallas to attend the Mad Hatter party my girlfriends threw for me. And Two wasn't the only surprise I was to have that weekend. A dear friend who lives in Payson, Arizona, about ninety miles away, called to say she was having car trouble and wouldn't be able to attend.

The night of the party, I'd been at the friend's house where the party was held for less than ten minutes, when I heard my Payson friend's distinctive voice over the clash of fifteen other women. Apparently, another friend hadn't been satisfied with the excuse of a broken car. She'd driven the one hundred eighty mile round trip, and would deliver my Payson friend home at the end of the weekend. Didn't I tell you my girlfriends are awesome?

Sixteen women attended that party, wearing a diverse collection of headgear. With family members from out of town contributing as well, seventy hats were presented to cover my soon-to-be bald head. They ran the gamut from a ridiculous turkey hat to a sophisticated confection that would have looked at home at the Kentucky Derby. I would never be able to wear them all, and eventually my granddaughter and I packed up the bulk of them to deliver to a facility downtown, which caters to breast cancer victims.

And so I walked into the oncologist's office the morning of December thirteenth, as prepared as anyone can be for something they don't really want to do, and said to the receptionist, "I'm here for chemo."

12/13/07...9am.

Well, Dad, today's D day - make that C day. I'm pretty calm at the moment. Maybe I'm just blocking. I'm getting pretty good at that. Or maybe the Lord has laid His hand of peace on my heart. I prayed the Lord's Prayer a few minutes ago in your name and mine. This morning I wasn't sure what to pray. That seemed right.

So, in a few hours I'll know. That's been weighing heavily on my mind. The not knowing what's going to happen. I didn't dare read up on it. I'd rather go into it with a form of trust rather than a book knowledge. Eight-A should be here in a couple of minutes. I'm glad she'll be with me.

I love you, Dad. I'll try to make you proud and deal with this with the grace you always showed. I'll tell you how I did later.

I won't bore you with the details. Chemo sucks, but it's doable. I will tell you that I began chemo on December thirteenth and when all was said and done at the end of March when I finished, I had lost all my hair, I could barely get up off the couch, and I looked like a World War II refugee—but I never threw up. The medications they have now are so much better than even five years ago.

I'll also tell you that December nineteenth was the worst day of treatment, the worst day of my life.

By that morning, I was feeling so bad I couldn't concentrate. Part of it was fear that I hadn't yet reached the worst point. I wasn't sure how much worse I could feel and still survive. I'd tried to pray my way through it, but couldn't even do that. Not knowing what else to do, I called Two. She was at work but didn't hesitate when she heard my voice on the line.

Thanks, Two. You'll never know what that meant to me.

We prayed together that morning and I survived. Now, I'm not a doctor. I don't even play one on TV, so I won't bother getting technical, but I soon learned the pattern of dropping blood counts and on consequent treatments, I didn't wait until I'd reached my worst point. My sisters and I shared seven conference calls the day before my counts hit bottom and headed off the worst of it in prayer.

He will cover you with His feathers, and under His wings, you will find refuge. Psalm 91:4

Chapter Eight

Doesn't Radiation Cause Cancer?

(Because that's what you're treating me for, you know?)

March ended finally and with it, I endured my last chemo treatment. Talk about red-letter days! I can't tell you how good it feels to know the worst is behind you. I still had radiation to face and reconstructive surgery, but nothing could compare with those four months of chemo.

I met the radiation doctor in late March. I'd scrambled my way through four months of hell with a minimum of tears, but for some reason, sitting in that waiting room, I started to cry. I have no clue why. I'd survived being sick as a dog, and weak as a kitten. I'd handled having my hands and feet go numb, and my bones aching like I'd been run over by a truck. My vision had deteriorated, my intelligence suffered due to 'Chemo Brain', and I'd lost every hair follicle on my body. What did I have to cry about now that the worst of it was done?

Looking back now, I realize I was simply exhausted, but reasoning that out later didn't help me at the time. Unfortunately, they called me back before I had the chance to pull myself together. From the looks the nurses were giving me, I'm sure they thought I was falling apart. They set me up with a counselor right then and there. I felt like an idiot.

When I'd finally convinced the counselor I didn't need a support group, that I already had plenty of support, they let me meet with the doctor. My first thought when he walked in the room was, since when do they give twelve-year-olds medical degrees? I swear, the guy had pimples. I kept waiting for his voice to break.

He seemed to know what he was talking about, though, and what the hell? I'd come this far trusting the Lord would deliver me into competent hands. I wasn't about to stop now.

Because of the potential damage to the skin during radiation, it was decided the reconstructive expanders I'd had installed immediately after the mastectomies should be replaced with the final implants first. In I went for surgery number two. With that done, and after a couple of weeks of recovery, I began radiation.

With the exception of some skin damage and fatigue, which I was suffering under already, radiation was a breeze. Then, two weeks into treatment, I suddenly developed a horrible backache. When you've been diagnosed with cancer, the first thing you think whenever you feel some oddity in your body is, Oh, crap. I have a new cancer. Since the ache was in the vicinity of my kidney, I was pretty much convinced I now had kidney cancer.

When I went in for radiation that morning, I told the nurses I wanted to see the doc when I was done with treatment. You have to understand that before the diagnosis, if I had made that request of a nurse and was told it couldn't be done, I would have meekly made an appointment for another day and left it at that. This particular morning I discovered an odd side benefit of having cancer. I was no longer meek. I repeated that I wanted to see the doc and that if I couldn't see *him*, I'd be heading across the street to the oncologist when I was done there.

The doctor was waiting for me when I came out of the radiation chamber.

05/20/08...12:30pm
Hey, Dad.
The radiation is going okay. I have begun to have some issues with my skin but even that isn't so bad compared to chemo. Everything is relative. If it weren't for my wacko emotions these days, the radiation treatments would hardly even be a blip on my radar. My odd emotional reaction doesn't make a lot of sense, but for some reason I find myself fighting tears more often than I would have expected, considering the process is so non-invasive.

Just the other day, a woman I have seen in the clinic a few times and have spoken to only once was coming out of treatment as I was going in. She carried a fistful of brightly colored balloons and announced with a smile, "It's my last day! They give you balloons when you finish." I congratulated her and felt genuinely happy for her, but a moment later, when she'd disappeared around the corner, I found myself about to burst into tears. I have no idea why.

I swear, Dad, there is something in the building that makes my hormones go mental, because I have had to fight tears at least five or six times in the couple of weeks I have been going there.

I asked the doc about that backache today. Okay, so now I have shingles. What the hell is up with that? When the nurse commiserated about this being just what I needed to hear, I told her that these days I wouldn't be surprised if an arm just spontaneously fell off.

My body suddenly has a mind of its own and seems to have turned on me. But, I'd rather have shingles than a tumor in my kidney, so that's something.

I met so many kind and pleasant people over the course of my treatment and the crew of radiation techs was no exception. For six weeks, they greeted me each morning when I arrived at the clinic for my daily dose of gamma rays. As I lay on the table looking up at a soothing country sky scene, complete with trees and puffy white clouds, they'd line up the huge machine that sent radiation into my right breast and shoulder. One day I commented on how strange it was to be having something that could potentially cause cancer aimed at my body, in an effort to cure me of cancer. The techs laughed, saying they'd heard that before. I commented that over the course of the eight months I had been treated for cancer, I'd had toxic chemicals and radioactive materials poured into me. I was beginning to think they pounded so many cancer causing materials into us cancer patients so that when we got it again, we wouldn't know who to sue.

They didn't laugh at that. I wonder why?

Chapter Nine

Yes, I Can Pick Up My Boobs

(Reconstructing the Ta-Tas)

I find it surreal that *I* have a plastic surgeon. I'm just not the type of woman who would ever consult one under normal circumstances. Yet, I've seen one. For nearly a year, I schlepped to his office, and marveled while he worked his magic.

How does one go about finding a plastic surgeon when they don't really want one? This, at least, was easy. There was only one plastic doc who had operating privileges at the hospital where the mastectomies were done, so the decision was pretty much made for me. Just the same, I went to meet with him. I don't know what I would have done if I hadn't liked him. Thankfully, I did.

11/1/07...4:45PM
Well, Dad, I met the plastic surgeon today. The whole experience was surreal. You should have pushed me to go to school to be a plastic doc. They obviously do well. Eight-A and I sat in his office feeling like a couple of Beverly hillbillies. You should have seen the place. It looked like the lobby of the Bellagio in Vegas. But with an office like that, he must be good. That relieves my mind at having only the one choice of reconstruction surgeons.
So, we have our schedule. Let the games begin.

After mastectomies, there are several choices of how to deal with the aftermath. If reconstruction is your choice, there are several different procedural options. Prosthetics are another option, and of course, one can always choose to do nothing. I chose reconstruction.

For about a half second I considered the option where they stretch tissue up from your stomach muscles to build breasts, but only because the doc said it was like having a tummy tuck, and hey, I was in my forties. What forty-something woman wouldn't benefit from a tummy tuck? In the end, I chose the procedure that seemed the least invasive.

My reconstruction began immediately following the mastectomies. While I was still on the table, my plastic surgeon inserted expanders where my breasts had been. Well, technically, they were tucked beneath the muscle of the chest wall. I looked like Arnold Schwarzenegger for a while. The expanders are temporary implants, filled over time, slowly stretching the muscles under which will go the final implants. Six chose the same procedure.

I don't know what I expected of this process, but the ultimate outcome seemed to me to be a little swatch of silver lining in an otherwise horribly black cloud. Okay, they'd hacked off my breasts, but I was going to get a brand new set. Six felt the same way, and for her, this part of the experience was mostly positive.

I suppose I would have found it more positive myself if I wasn't also dealing with chemo and radiation at the same time. Being sick while dealing with further operations sucked. In addition, since coming out of surgery that first day, I've never been physically comfortable with the reconstruction process. In the beginning, I felt as though I had a band of steel around my chest. The sensation eventually eased some, but even now that I am done, the sensation of having foreign objects inserted in my chest never quite leaves me. For a long time, the feeling was a constant reminder that I had breast cancer—as if I needed to be reminded—but thankfully, that has begun to ease too.

Between chemo and radiation treatments, I had the surgery to insert the permanent implants. I thought I was finally beginning the long healing process. I should have known better. My plastic guy had told me we would most likely need to do some tweaking and sure enough, several months later, the muscle on one side had broken down. In I went for a second set of implants.

About that time, we found out that a cousin of ours had been diagnosed with breast cancer as well. She is in her early fifties. Infiltrating Lobular Carcinoma again.

Six immediately had genetic testing done.

So, there we were, three daughters from our clan with breast cancer and all going through reconstruction at the same time. While my heart bled for my cousin, I had to admire her courage. Like Six, she handled her diagnosis with grace and strength, and more than a little bit of humor. The day she emailed to say she'd booked her appointment for her final surgery, I could only laugh at her excited anticipation of having her 'Tupperware Bowls' removed at last. I knew how she felt. I'd been *thrilled* to have those expanders removed.

All three of us have had a few laughs at the intensity of our individual plastic surgeons. They are artists, you see. The art of rebuilding a breast where none exists isn't an exact science, but these guys are constantly striving for perfection.

With the three of us all but done with reconstruction, we planned a family reunion. Mom was turning eighty and a weekend was planned in St. Louis, where our cousin lives and Mom had grown up. We were all excited to get together, especially Six, who couldn't wait to show off her new boobs. We knew she was pleased with her results when she suggested the three of us have a wet T-shirt contest while we were there.

Yeah. Like *that* was going to happen.

Since the nipples of both breasts were removed during the mastectomies, I was nipple-less. Now that I was beginning to feel better and I had my second set of new breasts, I was anxious to be finished with reconstruction. Having nipples represented being finished in my mind.

Truthfully, lacking nipples wasn't an issue for me. I didn't, and still don't, think of my breasts as breasts anymore. They look like breasts, sort of, but really, they're just numb bumps. Any nipples I would eventually have 'attached' would be for vanity and aesthetics alone, but though I couldn't have cared less, I wanted to look as normal as possible for my husband.

With the family reunion looming, I sat in the chair in the plastic surgeon's office. I was there to have the stitches removed from the last surgery, and my sense of humor reared its quirky head. I asked him what kind of time frame we were looking at until I could finish up with the nipples. He explained that I still needed to heal a bit more before we could proceed.

"Not that I'm in a hurry," I said, "but you know about my sister and cousin. I'll be meeting up with them in June and my sister has a wet T-shirt contest planned for the three of us."

He stood there looking at me, his eyes narrowing slightly. I could practically see the gears of his professionally competitive nature engage before he said in all seriousness, "I can make sure you win that contest."

I laughed like a loon.

Two weeks later, I happened to be changing clothes in front of a mirror and saw what looked like a dime sized, blood blister at the center of the incision on my right bump. The right side is where I'd had radiation and my first thought was, what now?

I called the plastic doc and left a message, but then called back again when my daughter-in-law looked at it and said, 'Mac, that isn't a blood blister. That's your implant!"

Because of the skin damage caused by radiation, the suture from the last surgery hadn't held, tearing apart to expose the implant beneath. By ten that morning, I was booked for emergency surgery. I'd already spoken to the doctor, the hospital, and my insurance company when the phone rang. The call was from my plastic guy's office assistant.

"We have a problem," he said.

"What's that?"

He went on to explain that the implant contact at the hospital was on vacation, so he hadn't been able to procure the implant I would need. They had some on hand at the office, but with the doc in surgery all day, he wouldn't be returning there before meeting up with me. His assistant was the only one in the office, so there was no one else available to deliver my new implant across town.

"So, you want me to come get the implant?" I asked.

"I can't believe I'm asking this, but yes. Would you mind?"

I could have said no, and let a courier deliver it, but hey, how many women can say they've driven across town with their boobs in the passenger seat? So, I walked into the hospital with my new implant and two spares under one arm.

"What have you got there?" the registering nurse asked as he led me back into pre-op.

"I picked up the implants from the doc's office."

"There are three in here," he said confused, looking in the box.

"Yeah, well," I said. "I think the doc is planning to make me into a Picasso."

Sometimes you just have to laugh.

Chapter Ten

Where Would You Like Your Nipple?

(Are we there yet?)

If you've recently been diagnosed with breast cancer, you'll soon be faced with some of the most important decisions of your life, all while you are at your least capable point emotionally. I wish I had a solution for this dilemma. I simply don't.

All I can suggest is that you do what I did. Asking the Lord to guide me in my decisions helped me tremendously. If you don't know Him, don't worry. He loves and hears us all. This illness will bring you to your knees. While you are down there, why not ask for His help?

In addition, ask a lot of questions of the professionals, and don't let anyone force you into making a decision before you are ready. Though it may not seem so, delaying a decision for a day or two won't change your outcome.

Along with the big, scary decisions, there will be many small and medium ones. For me, many of them fell into the bizarre category as well.

Finally, I was deemed healed enough to begin the process of getting my nipples. As if that sentence itself isn't bizarre enough on its own, a perky, twenty-something assistant joined me in one of the expensively decorated rooms at the plastic guy's office. Slim and sleek, she stood next to me in front of a large mirror, blonde perfection in professionally tailored scrubs. Naked from the waist up, I stared at our contrasting reflections, feeling like Carol Burnett at an R-rated beauty contest.

"Where would you like your nipple?" the assistant asked.

Another red-letter day.

To some of you, that probably sounds like a very important decision. However, to me, it was just another ridiculous moment in the new normal of my wacky world. It took me exactly three seconds to put a finger to the center of my nipple free bump and say, "Here?"

An hour later, I had a nipple. Freakin' wild! Again, I won't bother explaining the process as each doc has his own way of doing it. Since then, I've had the second nipple 'installed' and while they can't really be considered nipples by any stretch of the imagination, I'm content with the results. Next on the agenda - tattoos. Yes, that's right. We reconstructive chicks get to have areola's tattooed. And that is just one more ridiculous statement I never expected to come out of my mouth.

As I write this, it has been five years since I found the lump and my life changed. It's been a long and arduous adventure. I've experienced a range and intensity of emotions I never expected to experience, and if you've received a similar diagnosis, you will as well. You'll know disbelief and fear, anger and frustration, but if you are lucky, you'll also know humor and hope.

Yes, being diagnosed with breast cancer is devastating. Yes, it's frightening and the treatments are horrendous. But with new advances coming along all the time, the treatments are also becoming ever more effective with each passing year.

My life has changed, but not all of the changes in my life have been negative. Facing this kind of illness strips you down to the bare bones of life and forces you to focus on the important things. In my case, that was a positive development and has ended up being an unexpected blessing.

Each horrible moment connected with my diagnosis and treatment was offset by a poignant moment with those I love.

Arriving home from the plastic doc's office one day, my granddaughter climbed onto my lap to lay her hand on my face. "Did the doctor make you all better now, grandma?" she asked.

That sweet little question cancelled out the discomfort of the muscle spasms caused by the expansion process.

"It'll be nice when you're done with all the surgeries and I won't have to worry about hurting you," my husband whispered to me one night.

That honest admission of his concern cancelled out the anxiety I carried that I wouldn't be physically attractive to him.

"Can I get anything for you before I leave, Mom?" my oldest son asked one day.

That gentle selflessness cancelled out the exhaustion I felt as I recovered from the latest round of chemo.

"We just called to see how you were feeling," my sisters said as I answered one of their many conference calls.

That camaraderie cancelled out the pity party I wanted to indulge in.

"I love you so much. I'm so glad you're going to be my mother-in-law," my then future daughter-in-law said as she wrapped her arms around me one night at a gathering of family and friends.

That loving touch cancelled out the nausea chemo left behind.

"You are one hot, bald chick," one of my friends teased when I removed my ever present hat while sitting down to dinner in a restaurant one night during chemo.

That silly taunting cancelled out the tears I'd shed as I'd stared at the clumps of hair gathered in the shower drain.

On the day I was to have my last radiation treatment, I awoke to find a bouquet of flowers and a note from my youngest son.

Mom, he wrote, *Congrats on your final day. I am so proud of you for staying strong throughout the entire thing. You may not know it, but you are such an inspiration to us all. Thank you for being the best role model in my life. I love you so much. I can't wait to see you healthy and happy. Love you, Mom!*

That single sheet of paper cancelled out all of the frustrating insurance paperwork involved in healing me of cancer.

Over the last five years, I've experienced many such poignant moments. Concentrating on those moments instead of the trials of treatment helped to keep me in a positive frame of mind, but more importantly, focusing on those moments allowed me to feel victorious, one step at a time. And with each tiny victory, I found myself closing the gap between victim and survivor.

I'm a different woman than I was in September of 2007. I've faced physical challenges I wouldn't wish on my worst enemy, and experienced emotions I never even knew existed. Physically, I'm different, but more importantly, battling breast cancer left me emotionally stronger than I ever thought I could be.

I'm not saying there won't be bad moments. There will be plenty of them. I still have them occasionally. The breast cancer adventure doesn't end with the completion of the initial treatment, but we live in an age where each day dawns with the possibility of incredible medical advances. In my case, my special ops commando is always on the lookout for new weapons in my battle for survival.

In that vein, I just recently completed a brand new preventive treatment to increase those crappy survival numbers I was given. Instead of the mid fifties, my numbers now stand in the low seventies. Yeah, baby! As I have, since the diagnosis, I will continue to fight my own personal battle using every tool in the medical industry's vast bag. God has placed some very smart people in my path who have and will continue to play a big role in my victory.

As of today, I am cancer free and with each new day, I regain more of the strength I lost over the course of treatment. Unfortunately, recurrence or the onset of a new cancer sometime in the future is an unpleasant possibility in my new normal, at least, as far as the medical profession is concerned. They work from their numbers. I'll continue to work from God's.

But, either way, dealing with the long term possibilities, as well as the day-to-day trials of cancer, is infinitely more palatable when you begin each day as a victor rather than a victim.

Since my diagnosis, I've met hundreds of women who have gone before me, and many of them faced this disease without the incredible medical and technical advances we have at our disposal today. They've been where I was five years ago, where you are today, and yet they are living full lives, quite often with renewed purpose. They are raising their kids, pursuing careers, and speaking out in the community.

If there is one common characteristic I've seen in all the survivors I have met, it is strength.

If you are just beginning your walk through this frightening disease, you probably don't feel strong. Don't beat yourself up if that is the case. You'll get there. Remember that everything they throw at you is doable. Take cancer vacations as often as possible, and stop to smell the roses while you're at it. Allow yourself to take things one-step at a time, and try not to stress over what comes next. It will come whether you stress over it or not.

Try Scarlett on for size. She not only dressed well, she was a smart woman.

He will cover you with His feathers, and under His wings, you will find refuge. Psalm 91:4.

Whether you know Him or not, God knows and loves you, and hears your pleas. His lap is always available.

So, close your eyes, breathe deep, and take that first step toward conquering the abyss. I'm dancing on the other side. I'll see you there.

Mac

***

About the Author:

I'm a wife, mother, and grandmother. My husband and I were blessed with two rambunctious little boys who we managed to raise into wonderful men without any disfiguring mishaps. Dirt bikes and ESPN are the order around our house, and life at the 'Testosterone Ranch' more closely resembles one of today's wacky reality shows, than yesterday's *Leave It To Beaver*.

A love of books, specifically the romance genre, has been a lifelong affair, both as a reader and a writer. My bout with breast cancer sharpened my resolve to see my stories shared with others. As of today, I am a five-year survivor, living my dream.

Discover other titles by Mackenzie Crowne at Amazon.com or visit me at my home on the web @ mackenziecrowne.com